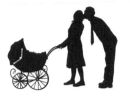

WHAT HAPPY PARENTS DO

Also by Carol Bruess and Anna Kudak

What Happy Couples Do
Belly Button Fuzz & Bare-Chested Hugs—
The Loving Little Rituals of Romance

Ninety-Three Cents and a Little "Humpty Dumpty"

WHAT HAPPY PARENTS DO

The Loving Little Rituals of a Child-Proof Marriage

Carol J. Bruess, Ph.D. & Anna D.H. Kudak, M.A.

Published by Fairview Press, 2450 Riverside Avenue, Minneapolis, Minnesota 55454. Fairview Press is a division of Fairview Health Services, a community-focused health system, affiliated with the University of Minnesota. For a free current catalog of Fairview Press titles, please call toll-free 1-800-544-8207. Or visit our Web site at www.fairviewpress.org.

Library of Congress Cataloging-in-Publication Data
Bruess, Carol J., 1968-
    What happy parents do : ninety-three cents and a little "Humpty Dumpty":
    the loving little rituals of a child-proof marriage / by Carol J. Bruess & Anna Kudak.
        p. cm.
    ISBN 978-1-57749-177-4 (alk. paper)
    1. Marriage. 2. Married people. 3. Parents. 4. Communication in marriage.
    I. Kudak, Anna D. H., 1982- II. Title.
    HQ734.B9133 2008
    646.7'8--dc22
                          2008010050

Printed in Hong Kong
First Printing: August 2008
12 11 10 09 08   5 4 3 2 1

Interior design by Natalie Nowytski, Renaissance Jane
Cover illustration by Corbin Frost

For my parents, "Beangrinder" and "Bunka,"
who model the best of both parenting and partnering
—Carol

For my parents, "Debbie Lynn" and "Johnnie Joe,"
who taught me how to love the rain
—Anna

The Loving Little Rituals
of a Child-Proof Marriage

Did you know that, for most couples, marital satisfaction dips significantly during the years of raising babies and young children? Were you aware that, for two thirds of couples, conflict and hostility increase dramatically after their first baby arrives? For almost all couples with children, emotional intimacy decreases and romance cools. If you have children—whatever their age—you are likely saying, "No kidding." But there is no need to despair. You *can* DO something to maintain or re-establish an emotional connection with your spouse after you have children. You *can* find more joy and intimacy with your partner during this time when other relationships are constantly trying to draw your attention away from your spouse. You *can* be more intentional about the ways you interact with your spouse and, by being more intentional, increase the happiness you are feeling in your marriage. How can you do this? That's what this book is about.

In this follow-up to *What Happy Couples Do*, we turn our attention to couples who stay happy and connected amid the poopy diapers and the T-ball car pools; who stay satisfied and in love while negotiating curfews and computer time with their teenagers; who carve out time for their marriage despite temper tantrums and the terrible twos. Is it possible for a couple to maintain their intimacy while still meeting the often overwhelming demands of raising children? Absolutely! As the stories in this book reveal, happy couples with children make sure they still DO things together, repeatedly and often. They find simple, playful, often private, but always significant ways to stay connected. They develop, maintain, and protect rituals created by and intended for just the two of them.

Research shows that one of the most important things you can DO for your child's health and well-being is model a happy marriage. John Gottman, the noted marriage researcher, has found that babies raised by unhappily married parents suffer not only emotionally but also intellectually. Babies of unhappily married parents are slower to develop speech, to learn to use the potty, and to learn ways to comfort themselves. In Gottman's words, "The greatest gift a couple can give their baby is a loving relationship." We couldn't agree more.

This book will teach you how to build, maintain, or resurrect a strong and loving marital relationship as your family expands. It will encourage you to develop loving little rituals—those predictable, steady, and soothing activities that can set and re-set the tone of a marriage. It will inspire you to cool your conflict and heat up your romance by developing durable and dependable ways of shifting your attention (however briefly) from your kids to each other. We've learned from the happy couples we talked with that when the going gets rough a few rituals can repair and restore a loving connection. We share with you here dozens of such rituals to give you some ideas about what you might try to incorporate into your own marriage.

Rituals strengthen and improve relationships. Unfortunately, it is easy to let them slip away under the pressures of parenting. Let the stories and lessons within remind you that you can DO something about your marriage. You can DO what happy couples with children do. Your marriage is up to you. Why not enjoy it?

Share Your Stories

If you are inspired by the stories in this book and have your own rituals to share, please tell us about them.

Visit **www.whathappycouplesdo.com** and click on *Share Your Stories*. We would love to hear what you are DOing to maintain a loving partnership while parenting. We also invite you to share stories of rituals involving other relationships in your life—with friends, family, coworkers, whomever. Or simply e-mail us:

Carol Bruess and Anna Kudak
carol&anna@whathappycouplesdo.com

1 Little Individual Boxes

On Sundays when our girls were young, ages four and six, we liked to sleep a little later. So I would put little individual boxes of Cheerios and sippy cups on the table with napkins, spoons, and bowls. And then I would put two small pitchers of milk in the refrigerator on a low shelf. We would tell the girls to let mommy and daddy sleep. Our six-year-old was in charge of pouring the milk and making sure her younger sister could get her straw in the cup. We'd tell them that we'd call them when we woke up. They were so good. We had a king-size bed, and my husband would yell at the top of his lungs, 'Girrrr-lllls!' He made two syllables out of one. You'd hear their little feet scamper up the stairs, and then they'd jump into bed with us and cuddle. It was an absolute joy. And we were rested and happy. A win-win.

To be healthy, your marriage *and* family both need to win. It's easy to nurture one at the expense of the other, but the cost is high if you do.

Find a way, no matter the age of your children, to make sure you and your spouse are happy in your relationship. If your marriage is not happy, your children are going to know it deep in their hearts and souls.

Those little feet that are scampering up the stairs now will soon be wearing shoes the size of yours. And they will undoubtedly reproduce— if not consciously, then in the actions of their own relationships—scenes like the one described on the opposite page. When they begin their own adult relationships, they will draw on a lifetime of moments from their child-hoods. They will recall with fondness the loving gestures of parents who nurtured and provided a safe place for each other as well as their children.

Do you want your children to have a healthy head start on happiness in their future marriages? If so, make sure yours is happy right now.

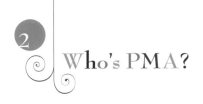

2 Who's PMA?

Frequently, after talking about the best and worst parts of our children's day, my husband and I will want to talk about things that happened to us at work that day. Because our children are getting more mature ears, we are very careful never to use the names of specific individuals at our offices. Instead, we use the initials of the person we are talking about. For example, if we are talking about Peggy Marie Anderson, we will have a conversation that goes something like: 'Whew. PMA was on a rant today.' It's a secret language that our kids are not privy to. Lately the kids—now between the ages of seven and twelve—will ask, 'Who is PMA?' We always simply say, 'Just somebody we work with.'

This couple is definitely onto something. That something, according to researchers, is the use of a secret language to forge a closer bond. A secret language allows a couple to share their thoughts, experiences, and feelings, even when little ears—or in-law ears—or neighborly ears—are listening.

In every relationship, but especially in happy marriages, there is a need for both openness and privacy, for revealing and concealing. Believe what the research shows, and create your own private language. DOing so will construct a loving boundary around your twosome. Why not GIAT? (Give it a try!)

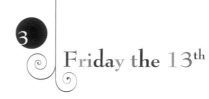

3   Friday the 13th

" Number thirteen is our lucky number. We were married on a Friday the thirteenth, and since then we have adopted the number thirteen as 'our' number. When it's the thirteenth of any month, we call it a special day. When we see a basketball or football player wearing number thirteen, we cheer extra loud ('He's playing for us!'). When a purchase totals thirteen dollars (and any cents), we smile at each other. Our kids point out the number thirteen to us, too. The number thirteen might be unlucky to others, but it's definitely not to us. We are more in love now after seventeen years of marriage than we've ever been ... and it all started on Friday the thirteenth. "

Culture is commonly defined as a group of people who share a set of values, beliefs, and history, as well as a common language, set of rituals, and symbols. Did you know that your marriage is a mini-culture, made up and strengthened by the language, rituals, and symbols you share? The unique words, phrases, activities, and traditions that have meaning only in your relationship help preserve, celebrate, and solidify your marriage.

As cultures preserve and celebrate themselves through the participation of their members in ritual and symbols, so do happy couples preserve and celebrate their marriage.

4 Theatrical Smooch

" *When Dad gets home from work, it can be a loud, happy, and determined contest to see which of the two kids can be the first to greet him. Yet, even with the deafening cries of 'Daaad,' Mom reigns victorious as the receiver of the first kiss. The kids may get to hug a leg and hang on for the ride, but Mom always gets the first, usually quite sloppy and theatrical smooch, followed by a lovely pinch on the tush (which, naturally, the kids find very amusing). Oh, and now that we have a dog, Dad's homecomings are even crazier and louder.* *"*

The happiest couples put each other first in their thoughts and feelings … and first in line for their lips! Even when kids, pets, and life demand your attention, make a beeline toward your spouse. You'll be glad you did. In the long run, your kids will be glad you did, too.

MAKE SURE YOUR
PRIORITIES ARE
IN ORDER.
KEEP YOUR SPOUSE IN
(1) YOUR THOUGHTS,
(2) YOUR HEART,
(3) YOUR DAY.

A Little Get Together

Sometimes, after my husband drops the kids off at school, he'll come home again for a little 'get together' (i.e. sex). He knows that I'm usually just starting to get ready for the day after they leave, so sometimes he'll even ring the front door bell. I answer the door and ask him what he is soliciting, and he responds by saying, 'You.' It's been our secret, fun way of staying intimately connected now that our children stay up past our own bedtime.

Without a doubt, couples are different after they have kids. They often lack the energy and enthusiasm for each other they fondly recall when they first were flirting, dating, and making love (every day!). But that doesn't mean that couples with kids can't or don't find ways of making time and crafting creative ways to stay physical, intimate, and affectionate. Sometimes it's as simple as a little "solicitation." Sometimes it's as tricky as scheduling time off work. Whatever it is for you, be sure to make time, again and again, for some "little get-togethers."

MARRIAGE
IS MUCH MORE
satisfying
WHEN YOU ↱SYNC↲
WITH YOUR SPOUSE.

I Do (Again!)

"Each year our church holds a dinner and service to honor all the married couples. It's a time when the couples attending renew their vows and reflect on their commitment to one another. We went the first year because some friends were going. Now we make a special effort to attend every year. It's the only time of the year that we both look deeply into one another's eyes and tell each other, out loud and in unison with all of the other hundred or so loving couples in the room, how much we love each other. It's a powerful way to reaffirm our partnership."

Renewing your wedding vows, whether you do it alone or with hundreds of others, is indeed a powerful way not only to say "I do" again, but, in essence, "We can!" and "We choose!" and "We are worth it." Think about how wonderful it would be to look each other in the eyes and say, "I am choosing you again."

DO something regularly to remind each other that your marriage is worth renewing and rejoicing in out loud—that your partnership is definitely worth every bit of effort you put into it. If you've never renewed your vows, why not do it this year, or even this month? Pick a day and make it happen. No need to wait for a "special" anniversary. Isn't your marriage special enough, right now, just the way it is?

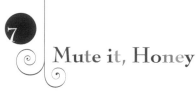

7 | Mute it, Honey

Sabrina and Carlos noticed their ritual of watching favorite television evening programs evolve over time to include one important rule: "Mute it" (the commercials, that is). Although watching their favorite shows is an activity they enjoy, they also cherish the intervals of time commercials provide to chat and catch up on the day after their children are in bed. So they developed the unspoken rule that commercials are muted. If one forgets and has possession of the remote, the other kindly but sternly says, "Mute it, Honey."

Happy couples often slip, without noticing, into a jointly constructed routine that meets both needs *and* interests. And that's a beautiful thing. Like so many couples who have children, Sabrina and Carlos have literally and intentionally found a way to quiet the external noise of daily life and create regular intervals for conversation.

Where is the "mute button" in your marriage? What do *you* do to quiet the noise—of cell phones, PDAs, children, extended family—so you can really tune into each other?

DO QUIET

THE EXTERNAL

NOISE

SO YOU CAN

TUNE IN

TO EACH OTHER AND

TO YOUR MARRIAGE.

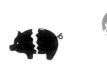

Was it 93 cents? Or 96?

I t's a question one couple uses to stop themselves before they start down a path towards useless arguing. They explain:

His parents constantly correct one another and bicker over the most trivial details—an obvious power conflict—which is unpleasant and embarrassing for all. Once they spent a whole evening arguing whether something had cost ninety-three cents or ninety-six cents. Using this phrase makes us laugh at ourselves and helps us restore proper perspective.

Maintaining or regaining perspective when conflict with your partner begins to spiral upward can feel impossible. Having a strategy such as uttering a short phrase or displaying a nonverbal signal—a phrase or signal that has meaning for only the two of you—can help.

Use something from your past to help you deal with problems now. What word, phrase, or gesture might be helpful at times when you're both losing perspective?

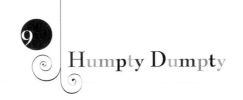

Humpty Dumpty

Marriage researchers agree that physical intimacy is an important aspect of the marital relationship. It may not surprise you to learn that many couples develop a private language for intimate matters (sexual intercourse, body parts, personal hygiene, sexual feelings). Such language serves important functions, allowing couples to talk more openly about potentially difficult or taboo topics. It also allows them to talk or make requests even when their children are present or there are similar constraints. So, if you're looking for a way to ease tension or personalize private matters, take a look at how other couples have developed their own intimate language. Consider how having a unique way to talk about sex might be a better (or more fun) way to go about it:

Requests for Sex

"Let's do the 'Humpty Dumpty.'" "Want to take a porking?"
"Let's play twister." "Let's go skiing."
"Let's have ice cream." "Let's get together."
"Let's get dog knotted." "Com-mon."

"Wanna take a nap?"

"Wanna noogie?"

"You wanna?"

"Wanna make a movie?"

"You want dessert?"

"Let's nookie."

"Let's have a party."

"Let's lube the chasis."

Raising the eyebrows

Tickling the palm

"Wanna little?"

"Wanna P.H. adjustment?"

"Let's do the twist."

"Hey … the kids are gone."

"Let's water the flowers."

"How about a twizzler?"

"It's picnic time."

"Let's play games."

"Is Herbie going to meet
     Alice tonight?"

"Let's get some bread and butter."

"Walter's [Wilma's] lonesome."

"Want to 'oh baby?'"

"Let's play checkers."

"I need to make an appointment."

"Let's sauce."

"Purrrrrrrr."

"Kids, it's your bedtime."

"Frank wants to go swimming."

"Do we have a date tonight?"

"Let's snuggle."

"Hey hammer, wanna leg?"

"Let's play peek-a-boo."

"Let's get a movie."

"Let's take a ride."

"It's love bug time."

Terms for male and female body parts (you decide which are which):

Virgil	Peppy
Reggie	Alfred
Henry	Jack
Henrietta	Gus
Clookey, Super Clookey, and Pokey	Gracie
	Poo
Honey Pot	Ace
Huge	Peeper
Mr. D	Chiquita
Chickie	Herman
Junior	Big Daddy Rabbit
Rabbit	USDA choice

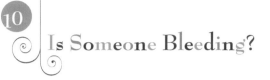

Is Someone Bleeding?

At the end of a workday we spend a minimum of fifteen minutes in a room away from everyone else to catch up on the events of the day. With small children under foot and the need to discuss our adult lives, we shut the door and tell them, 'Don't bother us unless someone is bleeding!'

DO find your own system for staying connected with your spouse and catching up at the end of the day. Even five or ten minutes can make a big difference. If the tires on your marriage are feeling a little flat or you've noticed that you frequently need a bit of revving up at a certain time of day, invite your spouse for even a brief conversation behind closed doors. The great thing about mindfully attending to the transitions of the day is how the moments that follow flow more peacefully and calmly. And so will your marriage!

Wife Unit #29

We have a nickname for each other that we use on a regular basis when we're feeling good about each other. I call him 'husband unit number one,' and he calls me 'wife unit number one.' But when we're angry, we increase the number to reflect just how mad we are. I might call him 'husband unit number 34,' or, if I'm really mad, 'husband unit number 157!' The increase in number is a clear indication of just how mad or upset we are. It really works.

For many couples, it's hard to know how to express displeasure—and do it constructively. Take a cue from the couple above who has developed a smart, creative, and very precise idea: an "anger barometer," which gives each spouse the chance to identify in numbers just how unhappy he or she is at that moment.

What's your marriage barometer? Do you have a constructive way to let your spouse know his or her "number?" If not, consider developing a way to reduce defensiveness while increasing expressiveness.

DO DEVELOP
A SYSTEM
FOR REDUCING
DEFENSIVENESS
WHILE BEING OPEN
TO *expressiveness*.

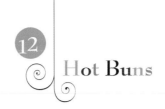

12 Hot Buns

My husband and I have a little joke about the heated seats in our car. We often find ourselves whispering this joke to each other when our kids are in the backseat. Because we live in a cold climate, heated seats are a must-have. When we get in the car, he'll turn on the seat heater, then lean over and whisper, 'How hot would you like your buns?' I'll say, 'Isn't it hot already?' Then he'll say, 'Ain't no seat gonna make yours any hotter than it already is. Your seat is as hot as it can get, honey.'

Let's just say that whether your spouse empirically has hot buns or not, telling him or her so surely *can't* hurt.

13

Playing with Produce

We go grocery shopping together on Friday nights, sometimes late after a date night out. We'll often be the only ones in the store, just playing around with the produce. It's great not only to accomplish something, like buying groceries, but, more important, to have some time for just the two of us.

Marriage is what you make it. Why not turn tasks and errands into opportunities to make a connection? Why not make the *ordinary* (picking out veggies and buying cereal) into something *extraordinary* (making the most of even the most mundane moments together)?

MARRIAGE IS WHAT
YOU MAKE IT.
INSTEAD OF ordinary,
WHY NOT MAKE IT
EXTRAORDINARY?

At That Very Moment

*"   On November 11, 2001, at exactly 11:11 a.m., my husband
(he was my boyfriend at the time) and I were driving in the car
when he asked what the date and time was. When I asked why
he wanted to know, he simply smiled and told me that someday I
would know why. Three years later, shortly after we had become
engaged, he told me that it was at that very moment—11:11 a.m.
on 11/11—that he knew he wanted to marry me, that we would
be husband and wife some day. Since then, almost every day, we
call or e-mail each other at 11:11 a.m. (or kiss at 11:11 p.m. if
we're still awake) to say 'I love you.' If we can't call at that time,
we try to stop wherever we are and quietly, by ourselves, take a
moment to remember how much we adore each other. "*

Are you willing to take a moment out of every day to remember and acknowledge how much you adore your spouse? If you aren't currently doing this, pick a time. How about 1 p.m. before your busy afternoon gets underway? Or 9 a.m., so you can begin the day lovingly? Or maybe 2 p.m. is when your wedding ceremony started many years before (and now the time your baby's afternoon nap begins). The important thing is that you commit yourself to reaching out to your spouse every day and saying, "I love you." You probably already realize that DOing this simple gesture produces anything but simple rewards.

MAKE THE TRANSITIONS
IN YOUR DAY MORE

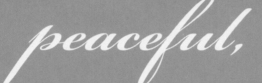
peaceful,

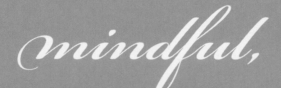
mindful,

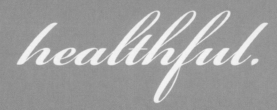
healthful.

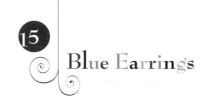

Blue Earrings

I have a pair of blue earrings. When I wear them, my husband knows that I've had a really bad day, that I'm in a bad mood, and that he should probably give me some extra space. This has greatly reduced the need for my husband to say, 'Ah, if I had only known....'

If you knew in advance that your spouse had faced problems and challenges during the day, would you treat him or her differently? With more kindness? With more patience? Marissa often wished her husband Todd could better anticipate her needs, especially at those times of the day when their kids demanded so much of her attention. So she came up with the blue earrings as a way to silently let her spouse know how she was feeling. Using this symbol reduced the need for conversation when what she really wanted was time to decompress and be alone with her thoughts.

What kind of secret code could you and your partner use to let each other know what you're thinking, needing, or wanting? How might you reduce the number of times you need to say "Ah, if I had only known..."?

Ten Miles or Less

When we're riding in the car, we both know what the other means by asking, 'How are you doing?' The answer is not an explanation, adjective, or even a sentence; it's simply a number. Because we often take long driving trips for vacations and holidays, we have devised a system for indicating to the other exactly how bad we need to pee. We developed this code after once having a pretty serious miscommunication about the severity of a need to stop. Our code rates need on a scale of one through ten. We don't worry too much if the number is five or less, but after that, things get more serious.

__Six__ is an initial warning number, just a heads-up.

__Seven__ means it's time to start watching the signs and planning to stop at the next city.

Eight *means we need to stop in ten miles or less.*

Nine*, it is necessary we stop at the next bathroom we see.*

If you hear **ten** *then you'd better be on the next exit without question or someone is going to be cleaning up the car!*

The ability of couples to develop a creative system of symbols helps make marriage more exciting, personal, and safe. If you have an issue that is resulting in frequent miscommunication in your marriage, see if you can devise a system with your spouse for making discussion of that issue easier, more efficient, and more fun. Whether the issue is peeing, leaving a social event, picking up around the house, or dealing with some pet peeve, using a number, hand gesture, or pat phrase can be a good way to say a lot without having to say much at all.

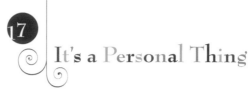

17 It's a Personal Thing

My husband and I have always agreed that if we're out in public or if our children are with us, no matter how mad or disappointed one of us is with the other, we will never let anyone else know. When we come home or find time alone, we then can let the other know. But we never bicker or argue in public or in front of our children because we believe it's disrespectful.

Have you ever had the chance to enjoy the creative spontaneity of an improvisational comedy group? Scenes evolve, change, and develop seamlessly, even though the performers work without a script. In improv, performers spontaneously act and react, making spur-of-the-moment decisions that are often brilliant and hilarious. Although the performance may appear random or chaotic, it's anything but. Improv artists follow a fixed set of rules to be successful, and they depend on their fellow performers to follow these rules as well.

Successful couples interact in similarly fluid yet structured ways. Like good improv, good marital communication is neither random nor effortless. Solid marriages are based on jointly developed rules that have emerged over time and clearly delineate what each partners can expect from the other.

Rules create the conditions for successful spontaneity. They help you and your partner better understand and anticipate what the other needs and wants. When this happens, you are more likely to respond to each other in productive and healthy ways, even in difficult times.

DO develop your own rules improvising on the stage of life. The result can be as brilliant as the artistry of the best improv performers: a seemingly effortless performance that you would be proud for anyone to see.

18

Dreaming of Dressers

"We like to go to a furniture store and select the most dreamy new bedroom furniture we can find. But we don't purchase it. We go just for fun. We pick out bedding, dressers, mirrors, and bedside tables. We even go so far as to ask about shipping costs and availability. But we never buy. We just pretend and dream. It's something we've always done. We get a huge kick out of it."

Pam and Ryan are working parents who find it challenging (to say the least) to enjoy time alone. To create more alone time for themselves, they schedule days off together. During one of those days off, their ritual of dream-shopping for furniture was born.

Although Pam and Ryan's window shopping is a fun and meaningful shared event for them, most marriage researchers would agree there is a more poignant lesson to be learned from what they are DOing here. More than just envisioning and dreaming about their ideal bedroom set, they are envisioning their future together.

Envisioning success is a powerful cognitive tool in almost any context (running a marathon, managing a conflict, even getting through a tough dental procedure). When you envision and dream with your spouse, the results can be even more powerful: you can create for yourselves a more solid and satisfying future. When you dream together, you are writing a draft of the rest of your life. And because you're writing it together, you're more likely to revise it together should adaptation become necessary.

Do you and your spouse have a joint vision for your future? Or any chapter in it? What kind of ritual can you develop to encourage the dreaming and writing of your future together?

DEVELOP A
JOINT VISION
OF YOUR FUTURE.

¶ REVISE *as* NEEDED.
          ^

ENJOY WATCHING IT
COME TO BE.

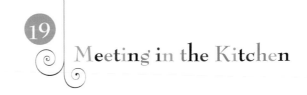

19 Meeting in the Kitchen

For the past thirteen years we've been meeting in the kitchen, right after the kids are in bed, to make four sack lunches together. I do everything except the sandwiches. Although it might sound boring and odd, I looked forward to this time of day. We are a team. And do you know how nice it is to wake up in the morning knowing those four sandwiches are made and those four bags are all ready to go? Amazing.

Have you ever stepped back to be amazed at the many routines you and your spouse have developed to make your lives better, more manageable, and more efficient? If you haven't, do so now. Stop taking these moments for granted.

DO take a moment to point out to your spouse, verbally or nonverbally, one way that you work well together.

20

Um, Honey ...

"We use the phrase 'Um ... Honey?' just before we provide honest feedback to each other about something the other is doing or not doing. For example: 'Um, Honey? Could you please not leave your clothes on the floor?' Or: 'Um, Honey? Would you mind making sure the garage door is locked when you're the last one in?' Or: 'Um, Honey? Could you be sure the kids' teeth are brushed BEFORE they go to bed?' We've used 'Um, Honey's' for the longest time because it helps us remember to be kind and considerate when complaining, making requests, or providing honest feedback about the other's behavior. It's been particularly important since having children—one of the most wonderful but also most stressful events of our marriage."

According to one of the most respected marriage researchers in the world, John Gottman, how you begin a conversation or conflict is the key to how it will turn out. Almost always, the first three minutes of a conversation or conflict will determine its outcome. Start softly and politely (using a simple complaint or observation), and the conversation is likely to continue that way. Begin with harsh criticism or sarcasm, and guess what? The conversation will most likely go downhill from there. Be aware that, over time, "harsh start-ups" predict divorce. DO find ways to begin and end your conversations kindly and respectfully. And toss in your own "Um, Honey..."—a simple phrase to soften your message. You, your spouse, and your kids will surely appreciate the results.

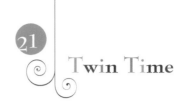

21 Twin Time

We have four children, the youngest of whom are twins. When the twins were infants, my husband and I would each take one for a 2:30 a.m. feeding. We would sit in a rocking chair every night in the babies' room and feed a baby. We didn't do this just to feed the babies, although they had to be fed. But the house was always so hectic when all the kids were around that we had no time to just talk alone. We really enjoyed the peace and quiet and time alone together, even if it was in the middle of the night.

It is often possible, though we don't always think about it, for a couple to transform a necessary chore, like awakening at 2:30 in the morning to feed a baby, into a cherished escape from the pressures of the day—a time for being together and present in the moment. How can you and your partner seize an opportunity to mold an already existing routine into a treasured and enjoyable ritual that provides a mini-escape? Even the briefest ritual can bring you a needed moment of intimacy, reassurance, or peace.

How can you and your partner *transform* an existing routine into a mini-escape?

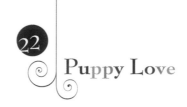

22 Puppy Love

"*Every night as we're heading to bed, and before we put Gracie, our new puppy, in her kennel for the night, we gather Gracie up in our arms, shout 'family hug!' and tell her how much we love her. We do love our puppy. But this is also a great way to make sure we hug each other every night, even when we're busy or exhausted.*"

Newlyweds Sandra and Brad are expecting their first child. They're already well on their way to maintaining a strong marriage after their new baby arrives by practicing rituals of connection like this—simultaneously demonstrating "puppy love" as well as affection for each other.

Committing yourself to a shared daily connection—one that is enjoyable, expected, and simple—can have resounding implications for your marriage. It is through such predictable rituals that two people create a shared reality. They create patterns that make their relationship distinct. They create a sense of certainty, acceptance, and affirmation.

So even if you're past the stage of "puppy love"—or aren't into family hugs with your pet—DO look at the predictable activities in your marriage and appreciate them for the comfort and love they provide day in and day out, every day, beginning and end. DO relish the fact that your patterns are like hugs—tender, warm, and wonderfully encouraging. And no matter how many children (or pets) you have, make sure that they are learning the most important lesson you can teach them: that their parents love and respect one another every day, in every way.

When you
nourish & respect
your marriage,
you are teaching your kids
the most important
lesson of their
lives.

Original Two-Pack

Now that our children are off to college, we can walk around the house naked if we want to. We have more freedom to be spontaneous. We might say, 'Let's go downtown and have some lunch,' or 'Let's go and—whatever.' We are more in tune with each other now. Looking back to when the kids were younger, we can see now that we should have devoted more time to just us instead of always worrying about the whole package.

If you have children, you can probably relate to the couple above. They have realized retrospectively that always focusing on their children ("the whole package") at the expense of their marriage (the original two-pack) was not a very good idea.

Decades of research support this realization. Those who nurture their marriage are significantly better able to care for "the whole package." And if one day you get the chance to walk around naked with your spouse to "go and—whatever," you might be very glad that you did devote some time for yourselves.

24 On The Porch

"I sit on the front porch to read a book or the paper late in the afternoon around the time my husband comes home from work. When I see him, I give him a simple wave and smile. It makes him feel good. And although we have never talked explicitly about this ritual, I know how comforting it is for me when he is standing on the porch as I pull up to the house."

Couples who have been married a long time or who have children that demand their energy and attention often find that a once warm and enthusiastic welcome-home greeting can disintegrate into a sideways glance, an impersonal announcement that a child needs to be picked up, or a brusque criticism: "Where have you been?" or "Why are you so late?" Think about how you greet your spouse, and ask yourself what kind of message you are sending to your spouse. Julia, in the example on the opposite page, did this and intentionally crafted a subtle welcome-home ritual for warmly and lovingly greeting her husband, Mark.

Even the least effort, such as merely being present and visible, can be a meaningful gesture in a life-long partnership, especially during that moment of the day when you reunite. What can you do to greet your partner more meaningfully? What small gestures might you already be making? Make note of them and continue doing them.

25 Something of Value

" One of our rituals is to buy things and fix them up.
We've bought many houses (always the cheapest house in a
neighborhood) and then worked on them. It takes a good deal of
time and effort, but we love it. Or we'll buy a used camper, and
we'll make it beautiful. Recently we spent thirty-seven dollars on
six bikes that we will refurbish. We love finding something of value,
stepping back and seeing how beautiful it could be, improving it,
and then passing it on. "

Is your marriage starting to buckle under the pressure of raising children? Has it begun to look and feel like a "fixer-upper?" If so, take a lesson from the couple on the opposite page. Step back from your marriage for a moment so that you can see its hidden beauty—the shiny core of your relationship, however tarnished it may have become by anger, criticism, routine, or apathy. Then DO something to begin to reveal its true beauty.

If your marriage needs a little fixing up, why not start today? Begin by polishing one little spot. Say one extra positive thing. Do one additional kindness. Give your spouse one extra smile.

Making even the smallest changes, and DOing so consistently over time, can make your marriage beautiful again. Even the most neglected and tarnished marriage can sparkle if you're willing to put a little bit of effort into fixing it up.

MAKING EVEN THE

SMALLEST

CHANGES CAN MAKE

YOUR MARRIAGE

beautiful

AGAIN.

26   A Monthly Mini-Celebration

For the last few decades Jill and Chris have acknowledged the day they said "I do" with a monthly mini-celebration they call their "month-iversary." They honor their June 6th wedding date on the sixth day of every month. These month-iversary celebrations are simple and, well, priceless. They have involved, for example, a handwritten note and a homemade cupcake. When the couple's children asked to be included in the cupcake eating, the couple simply responded, "Sorry, kids, you don't have a *honey-bunny* yet."

Do you want to wait an entire year to let your partner know that you cherish, adore, and appreciate him or her? If not, take a lesson from this happy couple: Create more frequent ways of celebrating each other.

27 Very Much Us

"When we celebrate something, we extend the celebration over at least two weeks. We did this before we had kids, and now we do it with them, or for our anniversary, and to celebrate any of our milestones as a couple. Like for my birthday, my husband will give me a little present every day for a week or two. We've even named it: It's called the Festival of Birthday. And it's not unusual for us to celebrate our anniversary with our friends, then with our children, then with our parents, and then with each other. Turning small celebrations into lengthy festivities is definitely something that is unique about us. Although some people think we're crazy, we wouldn't change it for anything. We love it. It's very much 'us.'"

It's not at all uncommon for couples and families to celebrate significant milestones such as birthdays and anniversaries. But what do you do to make your special occasions as a couple unique? Research shows that strong relationships are like strong cultures: they develop and maintain strong traditions. Your signature traditions—the unique ways you celebrate together over time —can have a more significant and profound influence on your relationship than you think.

This couple's ritual of stretching out their celebrations reflects a subtle but important aspect of their relationship culture that is uniquely their own, something they've committed to maintaining even after their family has expanded to include two children.

Whether it's a celebration or an everyday interaction, how can you make your traditions reflect something about your unique "us?"

DEVELOP AND PROTECT THOSE ACTIVITIES THAT REFLECT *YOUR* UNIQUE "US."

Wear and Tear

I give my wife children's books. Not for the kids, but for her. I'll get ones that have a message about us, like the book Guess How Much I Love You? *Or classics like* The Velveteen Rabbit *(about how we get better together with age and a bit of wear and tear). She might read them to the kids, but they are hers. She keeps them separate from the kids' books.*

Find a way to keep your marriage strong by taking care of each other. When your kids see that you are protecting and nurturing something (and someone) you love, they are much more likely to grow up and do the same. Don't make your spouse guess how much you love them. Show them with a book, note, or, better yet, by just telling them often.

No Arrow, No Sticky Note

"My husband gets up first, so he's the first one to see the newspaper. When I get downstairs to have breakfast with the kids, it's usually crazy. Someone's crying for cereal or over the wrong socks, so there's no time to talk. If there was something interesting in the paper, I'll know, because my husband will have left the paper open to that page. He doesn't circle the article. There's no arrow or sticky note. It's a game. I have to find it, and I always do. Sometimes it's a sad story about someone we know. Sometimes it's a depressing story about stock prices dropping at his company, or maybe a good review of a concert—someone we saw or he wants us to see. I like this ritual. It helps us stay connected in the crazy time we call morning with two little kids."

Life with little kids (or big kids, for that matter) can be a bit crazy. But happy couples don't let life get too messy, too sticky, or too stale. They don't allow themselves to get stuck. Instead, they create little games, invisible arrows that point out what they have in common, what they share, and what they know interests the other. Happy couples, over time, realize they must shift from "me" to "we." They nourish that "we" in even the smallest of ways, like the couple on the opposite page, who need no arrow, just an open newspaper on the kitchen table.

Note something that would pique the curiosity or nourish the interest of your spouse. Find a way to point it out. (Use an arrow if it helps.) When you do, you'll be giving something precious not only to your partner, but also to your partnership.

SHIFT FROM
"ME" TO "WE"
IN EVEN THE
SMALLEST
OF WAYS
EACH DAY.

30 Continue To Sit

With two small children, it's hard to find time to talk about adult things. So it has become our ritual to put the kids to sleep together. Once they have fallen asleep, we continue to sit in their room and talk about our day and the things that are bothering us. It helps to stay connected and feel that we are still close.

Our everyday talk composes our relationships. The way we greet each other, the way we say goodbye, the way we share our days, the way we ask things of each other. Relationships are built less on the big moments than on the everyday moments. Little by little, day by day, casual conversations construct and define a marriage.

Because your ways of talking with each other set the rhythms for and anchor your marriage, DO make sure you notice what your conversations look and feel like. If your conversations don't look and feel the way you think they should, change them. But first and most importantly, make sure that you are regularly setting aside time to talk.

As you look back on your marriage, what do you see? A legacy of richness, purpose, and meaning? Or a series of selfish acts and activities that have distanced you from your spouse?

According to researchers John and Julie Gottman (in their book *And Baby Makes Three*, 2007), happy couples with kids work thoughtfully and intentionally to create a family legacy and sense of shared purpose. A meaningful map helps them weather not only the often rocky transition to parenthood but also the years beyond. Solid, strong, and satisfied couples create a future of meaning and purpose for themselves (and their children) by looking back and asking questions about their values, beliefs, and family legacies.

So why not look back at your history? Then look at each other. What do you learn? What do you see? What choices are you making? DO something today. Make just one choice that will move you closer to the rich future you want for yourself, your marriage, your kids, and your family.

32 Squeeze Lightly

" When my husband and I were first dating (nearly twenty years ago), I told him that I loved the feeling of having the tips of my fingers squeezed lightly—a few seconds of firm but gentle pressure. When we are driving, he'll often take my hand and, one by one, gently squeeze each of my fingertips. It's something that reminds me of our past, a little loving gesture that shows me how much he remembers where our 'we' began. "

Little moments, light touches, and loving gestures are not insignificant. In fact, it is the accumulation of such little loving moments that creates a lasting marriage. Research on marriage has shown again and again that marriages are forged in the day-to-day, moment-by-moment, commonplace interactions of life.

It is through your rituals that YOUR MARRIAGE *is preserved, celebrated, and solidified.*

Anchor Down

"We both love to nap. When our kids were little, we would put them down for a nap (whether they needed it or not), and then we'd nap, too. In the summers, now that our kids are grown, our favorite place to nap is on our pontoon boat. We'll go out to the middle of a lake, anchor down, and nap. We used to float and nap but we once nearly took out someone's dock because we napped too long!"

Whether it's a nap, a jog, a drive, or a great dinner, reflect on what the two of you love doing and then make sure you always do it mindfully. Be fully present in the joy it brings you as a couple.

As the great mindfulness teacher and author John Kabat-Zinn reminds us (in his book *Wherever You Go There You Are*): "Sooner or later, the things you don't want to deal with and try to escape from … catch up with you." Many people have the romantic notion that if something isn't good here, it's certain to be better over there. If a job is no good, the next one will be better. If this spouse isn't working out, get a new one.

Instead of looking for greener grass elsewhere, happy couples simply enjoy their time together and, as a result, grow more together over time. They bask in the here and now, the bad times as well as the good times, and all the times in between. Happy couples learn very early that it's essential to carve out strategies for maintaining their favorite activities—or, as in the case of the couple on the opposite page, favorite napping spot. Happy couples enjoy their relationship as it happens. Pure and simple.

HAPPY COUPLES

GROW

IN THE

GOOD & BAD TIMES

AND IN THE TIMES

IN BETWEEN.

34 Hello, O Beautiful Husband

After our kids were born, my husband and I fell into that all-too-familiar pattern of being crabby with one another—taking each other for granted, criticizing each other, and simply not appreciating each other. We were so tired all the time and our kids demanded so much of our attention that we started to turn away from each other. When we finally noticed one day how cruel we had become to each other, we started doing something that has stuck to this day, more than fifteen years later. We now greet each other on the phone, in person, or by e-mail by saying, 'Hello, O beautiful husband of mine,' or 'Hi, O beautiful wife of mine.' This simple greeting reminds us daily how beautiful our marriage really is.

Kindness is contagious. Infect your marriage with it.

35
The Naked Debrief

"   My husband and I have a 'debrief' every night while we're on a trip. Well, mostly when we're on a trip visiting his parents or mine. Sometimes during the day we may both observe something ridiculous or annoying, and we'll look at each other and nod and realize that we have to let it go and put it on the debrief agenda. If we're staying in a guest room with twin beds, the debrief happens in one twin bed, and then it's right back to our own beds to sleep. The debrief is best when the other person didn't see something and you are sharing something new. Usually this bit of news is met with 'No—stop making stuff up,' to which the reply is, 'Seriously, why would I make this stuff up?' I love our debriefs. We're not mean. It's just a way of connecting at the end of the night, just the two of us, after a crazy day with our kids and extended families.

The debrief has assumed a variety of forms:

- *When he's traveling and I'm at home, I almost always get an e-mail debrief.*

- *Now that the technology is available to both of us, we often debrief in real time using instant messaging.*

- *After more than fifteen years of debriefing, we have added a 'pre-brief' before we leave or while traveling.*

- *My personal favorite: After returning from a trip, my husband has started calling me upstairs for a 'naked debrief.' As he says, "This gives a whole new meaning to the term "de-brief!"*

Happy couples know that to stay connected they have to make an effort to reach out to each other. Brief and debrief each other frequently about what's going on in your life. If you can work a "de-brief" in, all the better!

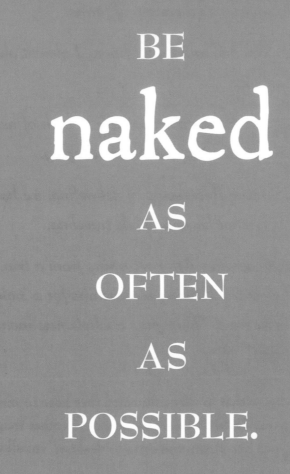

BE
naked
AS
OFTEN
AS
POSSIBLE.

36 By the Bathroom Bottles

My husband doesn't often purchase an extravagant gift for my birthday or our anniversary. (We've agreed not to over the thirty years of our marriage.) But he ALWAYS makes sure that he finds the perfect card and writes a meaningful, if brief, note inside. My favorite part is that he always has the card sitting either on my dresser or bedside table or by my bathroom bottles when I wake up on that special day. It's never just handed to me. It's always placed lovingly in a spot where I'll see it right away.

Lovingly. Isn't that the adverb that we would like to describe most of our marital interactions? "He lovingly welcomed me home." "She lovingly asked me about my day." "He lovingly remembered our anniversary. Again." Research clearly confirms that marriages where loving gestures outnumber non-loving gestures at least five to one work better and are happier. (See John Gottman and Nan Silver's *The Seven Principles for Making Marriage Work*.)

37 Our Private Stash

"My husband and I have a private stash of frozen cookie dough and ice cream that we hide in the bottom of the basement freezer. The kids have no idea it is there. After they go to bed, we often sneak down, sit on the floor, and eat our favorite treats in private. If we're really feeling brave, we'll even bring the treats upstairs to enjoy them at the table (hoping none of our kids is having trouble sleeping and comes down to find us). It's a great time for us to chat and connect, just the two of us and our favorite indulgences."

Every couple should have their secrets—their own private place, activity, or ritual. Whether the secret is what's hidden in the bottom of the freezer or what couples do on the sofa while praying those pajama-clad kids remain asleep, happy couples DO something to stay emotionally connected. Couples in strong marriages make sure that little moments of connection happen over and over. Such moments can make a huge difference in the long-term happiness of a marriage.

Think back to earlier in your marriage. What was your "private stash" or "favorite indulgence?" What did you do together that felt a bit secretive or sly—something you thoroughly enjoyed but didn't tell anyone else about (which of course made it all the more fun)? Then ask yourself what would happen if you revived your secret activity again? It couldn't hurt to at least try, could it?

38 Really Bad Wedding Video

"Every year on our anniversary we watch our wedding video. (Although we love it, it's a really bad video taken by my sister-in-law's dad.) After the kids go to bed, we put the video in and light the unity candle we used at the wedding. Then we laugh at our hair styles and the bridesmaids' dresses and cry when we see our grandparents, who have since passed away. Every year we seem to see something new in the Mass, which is fun. We notice that what we see is different as we grow older together."

According to respected marriage researcher and author William Doherty, being intentional about your relationship is essential to a strong, happy, and long-lasting marriage. This means consciously, deliberately, and continuously building a sense of connection. Doherty points out that happy couples need to be intentional about creating rituals of connection (watching your wedding video every year), learning about marriage (reading a book by a marriage expert and integrating new ideas into your daily life), maintaining a community of support for your marriage (dumping any friends who disrespect your spouse or your marriage), and setting boundaries for children (demonstrating that your marriage comes first by establishing rules that clearly say it is so). Doherty reminds us that if we are on automatic pilot as a couple we are likely to veer off course and lose track of where we're headed without even realizing it.

DO create and sustain rituals of connection. DO create an environment in your home and life that honors your marriage. You can avoid the bad in your marriage if you make an effort to do so.

DO CREATE

AN ENVIRONMENT

THAT'S

intentional & planful.

MAKE YOUR MARRIAGE

YOUR 1st PRIORITY.

A Trip Around the Lake

Our private place is our cabin. We go there almost every weekend. Although we are rarely there alone, we always take a trip around the lake in the boat, just the two of us. The kids think we are going sight-seeing, but actually we are using the trip around the lake to let go of the week and transition into the weekend.

Couples create a sense of who they are through their shared rituals. Any ritual—from the simple way the couple above transitions to the weekend to the most elaborately planned holiday tradition—can bind a couple closer together.

DO appreciate your rituals. Applaud yourselves for the stability, privacy, cohesion, predictability, and comfort your rituals and routines provide you. These interactions reunite you and your spouse again and again in the most lovely and loving ways.

40 Put it on the List

"After we had our kids, it seemed as if conflicts between my husband and me became tenser and more frequent. So, to help with this, we developed the phrase 'put it on the list.' When we're having an argument that doesn't seem to be going anywhere, we will say, 'Let's put it on the list.' The 'list' is imaginary. We don't actually have a list. It's just a way for us to end a conflict without actually having to resolve it. We feel better knowing we're 'putting it on the list' even if we never revisit it. If we do remember to bring it up again, it's more humorous, because we'll say something like, 'Remember that thing we put on the list last year?' It's also become a great way to avoid fighting in front of the kids. We can say, as the conflict is escalating, 'Let's just put it on the list.'"

Although it's not good to try to avoid all conflict in a marriage, postponing conflict until you are ready to deal with it (ideally, when you are feeling more connected) is positively OK. Not all conflicts need to be addressed immediately, especially if this means airing your troubles in front of your children.

Although "putting it on the list" might not be the right strategy for your marriage, DO identify what your strategy for managing conflict is. If you don't have a strategy, make one. If you do and it's not working, fix it or get a new one. There are as many productive ways to handle conflict as there are couples in the world. Find one that works for you.

41 Got My Flip-Flops On

"   *Getting ready for trips can be stressful. Doing the laundry and packing the clothing, supplies, and kids' stuff can be overwhelming. And it always seems that no matter how early I get started, my husband and I are still packing at midnight. The only thing that breaks the tension—and it works every time— is when my husband packs while wearing his flip-flops. He does this whether or not we're going to a warm vacation spot. I can come storming into our bedroom at midnight, arms full of swim diapers, sippy cups, clothes, shoes, and books, and there he is in his twenty-year-old flip-flops. He has a newer pair that he wears in warm weather and on vacation, but the old ones MUST be worn while he's packing. He always looks at me with a silly grin and says in a silly sing-song voice, 'Got my flip-flops on!' It works to keep the tempers and the blood pressures low.*"

Your marriage is a model for your kids. They will most likely base their future relationships off yours. Even your baby, if you have one, is taking note. Did you know, for instance, that a baby's blood pressure actually rises when the baby hears or sees his or her parents fighting? Imagine what your fighting does to the blood pressure of your toddler or teenager. Or yourself.

Take a cue from the couple on the opposite page. Find ways to maximize the humor during those times when you feel like minimizing (i.e., criticizing) the other.

FIND A WAY TO

MAXIMIZE

THE HUMOR

WHEN YOU ARE MOST

TEMPTED TO

minimize

AND CRITICIZE.

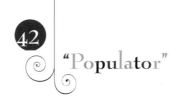

"Populator"

When I'm out, doing nothing in particular, I'll call my husband on his cell phone. He often will pick up and—in a voice that's low, smoky, and somewhat robotic but also somewhat sexy—say, 'Momulator.' And I, in reply, will say, 'Populator.' This started after we had kids (him 'populating' the earth). Prior to that I was simply Sugar Plum.

According to marriage researcher Judy C. Pearson (author of *Lasting Love*), happy couples tend to see themselves as extraordinary. She has found that the happiest of happy couples—those married forty or more years—look at their relationship through rose-colored glasses and refuse to take cues from the rest of the world about what they should or could be as a couple. They determine their own reality. Happy couples often distort, in a positive way, their relationship, experiences, and behaviors.

DO enjoy the beauty and comfort of your own reality as a couple.

Enjoy your own silly way of answering each other's calls. Greet each other with nicknames ("You are my populator"). Or simply enjoy the ease that comes with knowing someone for so long that your perceptions and expectations have become almost identical.

ENJOY THE
beauty & comfort
OF HAVING

YOUR OWN REALITY

AS A COUPLE.

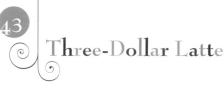

43 Three-Dollar Latte

" My husband and I are always in money-saving mode, trying to be conscious of our long-term financial goals. So, when gift-giving occasions come up, we try to be creative rather than spending a lot on things we don't need or even want. For instance, this past Valentine's Day morning I got out of the shower and was greeted by one of those three-dollar lattes our financial planners tell us to avoid buying on a daily basis. What a treat! Then, when I opened the garage door, I beheld my gleaming minivan. I had been complaining all week about how salt-encrusted it was, so Paul had taken it to the car wash. "

DO experience each moment, each emotion, each and every way you and your spouse are connected and coordinated. Consider the delightful way a car wash or cup of coffee can show respect and bring you closer. Such gestures honor both your partner and your partnership.

DO EXPERIENCE
EACH AND EVERY WAY
THAT YOU
AND YOUR SPOUSE
ARE *connected*
AND *coordinated*.

44 Apply Oxygen Mask

"*My husband grew up in a large family and learned early on that if you don't get your food quickly, there might not be any left. So now, when we're at a party or family function with the kids, I will often look over and find my husband already sitting down eating and visiting while I'm struggling with five plates of food for our children and me. It's rather irritating. So I'll say 'Apply oxygen mask first before assisting others' to remind him that there are other people who need help, too. We both laugh. It's become a phrase that often comes in handy.*"

DO make sure you create ways to laugh or insert a bit of humor when tensions rise between you and your spouse. According to marriage researchers John and Julie Gottman (*Ten Lessons to Transform Your Marriage*, 2006), if you can repair, you can avoid despair.

"Repairing" a conflict can take many forms—for example, spontaneously saying "I'm so sorry," flashing a grin or a smile, or, as the couple on the opposite page aptly demonstrates, developing a funny phrase that will cool the rising temperatures.

So many of us wait for our spouse to make the first move to repair a conflict. We get stubborn or selfish. Our minds build arguments and do negative mental acrobatics. But what if, even just once, you were the first to say, "I'm so sorry." Or, "Isn't this silly!" Or, "I'm such a fool for being so foul." You will probably be glad you did. And, over time, you may also be more likely to avoid what couples in too many marriages sometimes feel: the unwelcome and unnecessary feelings of despair.

DO:

Smile OFTEN.

APOLOGIZE.

MAKE JOKES.

ATTEMPTS TO REPAIR

WILL REDUCE DESPAIR.

45 Our Own Private Dance Party

We consider ourselves music geeks. Three or four times a year, after the kids are in bed, we have our own private dance party in the basement. We play music and dance like crazy. One of the best parts is taking turns playing DJ. One of us plays a song, and then the other plays a song. And we dance and dance. It's actually the only time I've seen my husband dance when he's not looking like he's kung foo fighting!

Dance. Laugh. Look like a geek. But don't care.

Only in a loving and trusting marriage can we do all of the above and still know, deep down and day after day, that the other will love us more and more. Without question or hesitation.

Ah, what a lovely thing marriage can be. DO be sure yours is as wonderful as it can be.

46

Real People Again

" *One of the things I appreciate about my husband is that he's a coffee drinker. I love coffee and drink a lot of it. Since having kids, we will sometimes—in the middle of the day if both kids are occupied—we'll get a cup of really good coffee. While we're sitting there, with our groovy little cup of European coffee, we'll be reminded of places we lived before we had kids. And even if it's just twenty minutes, I'll always say: "We're real people again. And I'm drinking coffee with a grown-up that I'm married to!"* "

It's amazing how little it takes, when you are parents of young children, to bring you satisfaction again. Yet so many of us deprive ourselves (and thus our relationship, our souls, and each other) of what actually infuses us with the goodness that will spill out toward and into our children and their futures.

DO make an effort to get that groovy cup of coffee with your spouse. Or whatever will remind you of what your relationship was, where it all began, and why you are creating this family you adore and cherish. You are married. You are grown-ups. DO something that will joyfully remind you of that.

47

A Little Island

"We built a small deck on the back of our house and bought a table and chairs. We sit there on weekends and have a drink or read the paper while the boys play in the backyard. And it's nice because we're set apart from the boys, and we can read, talk, or drink coffee while they play. It's nice to have our own little space, a little island. The reason we built it this way is so we'd have a area where we can sit and watch them."

Although giving lots of love and attention to your children is essential for their growth and development, having what Drs. John and Julie Gottman call a "child-centered marriage" is not a good thing at all. (Read more in the Gottmans' book *Ten Lessons to Transform Your Marriage*.)

Why? Because couples in child-centered marriages often neglect their marriage, putting their parenting responsibilities and their children's needs first. They favor these needs over nearly everything else. When, as the Gottmans say, your marriage (and everything else) takes a backseat to your children, you are missing the point.

DO build a little island around your marriage. Protect it and plant it with goodness. Out of your sacred and satisfying marriage will grow all the other gorgeous things you dream of: great kids, happy and fulfilling lives, and a loving family.

DO PLANT YOUR MARRIAGE WITH *goodness.*

THEN WATCH HOW *gorgeous* THINGS WILL GROW.

Learn
to handle
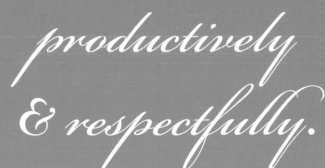
CONFLICT

productively

& respectfully.

Land On Your Face

"Our family is very competitive. My wife and I have the most fun when we're competing against each other (kids not included). It could be a game of cribbage. Or it could be a contest to see who can shoot a rubber band the farthest—or who can throw a pillow up, hit to the ceiling, and get the pillow to land back down on the other's face while we lie in bed at night."

Hold up a magnifying glass to your marriage and ask: What am I taking for granted in my daily interactions with my spouse? What can I do to be more mindful of the times, places, and opportunities in our lives? What can we do as a couple to fully embrace the current moments, pleasant or unpleasant, simply as they are?

DON'T JUST *ENDURE*
YOUR MARRIAGE.
MAKE EACH MOMENT
A *magical* ONE,
WHATEVER IT MAY BE.

49 Spousal 911

" My husband and I have developed a signal for getting in touch with one another during our busy workdays while our two kids are at school. He knows that if I call once on his cell phone, I'm probably just calling to say hi or to give him some news about one of our kids. Two calls in a row means I need him to call me. If I call three times in a row, it's the equivalent of a 911 call: Drop what you're doing, walk out of any meeting, and call me immediately! This signal has helped us be more responsive to each other. We feel freer to call during the day without worrying about interrupting at a bad time. There have also been times when we do need each other immediately—like when a kid is sick. It's so nice to know that we're there for each other when we really need to be. "

In happy marriages, couples are there for one another. Not all the time, but any time. Not every minute of the day, but, on some level, any minute of the day. Essentially, happy couples are best friends: They know they can count on each other when really needed—for both the big and the small, the little conversations and the big deals.

Do you and your spouse have a signal to let each other know when you need each other—when you really want to talk or have a desire for backup in your busy lives? If not, create your own 911 signal. Or follow the example of another couple who uses the phrase "I insist" for a similar purpose. This couple reserves the right to say "I insist" on those rare occasions when one of them feels especially strongly about something: a deep need for a decision to be made, an idea accepted, a request supported. "I insist" means: "The conversation is over. You must do this for me."

Whether it's "I insist" or 911, DO make sure your spouse knows that you will be there whenever, however, or why-ever he or she needs you.

50

My Kind of Fishing

One time, before we were married, my brother caught my husband-to-be and me in a fishing boat having a little 'alone time.' We were, to say the least, embarrassed! My brother yelled out, 'My kind of fishing!' Since then, my husband and I will often use that phrase as a private way to be playful in front of others or our children. Sometimes we even use it as an invitation to engage in a little 'fishing' later on.

Don't like fishing? Try the kind developed by the couple above. And know that using phrases that have meaning only for the two of you function like cement in a marriage, affirming a shared memory, bond, or experience. Whatever the saying, or whatever the shared memory, a word or two about it (especially when it makes no sense to others) is a sensible thing to have.

The
WILD & WONDERFUL
beauty
OF YOUR MARRIAGE
IS UP TO
YOU.

Bibliography

Buri, J. (2006). *How To Love Your Wife*. Tate Publishing.

Doherty, William J. (2001). *Take Back Your Marriage: Sticking Together In a World That Pulls Us Apart*. Guildford Press.

Gottman, J. M., & Gottman, J. S. (2007). *And Baby Makes Three: The Six-Step Plan for Preserving Marital Intimacy and Rekindling Romance After Baby Arrives*. Crown Publishers.

Gottman, J. M., & Gottman, J. S. (2006). *Ten Lessons To Transform Your Marriage*. Crown Publishers.

Gottman, J. M. & DeClaire, J. (2001). *The Relationship Cure: A 5-Step Guide To Strengthening Your Marriage, Family, and Friendships*. Three Rivers Press.

Gottman, J. M. & Silver, N. (1999): *The Seven Principles for Making Marriage Work*. Orion.

Kabat-Zinn, J. (2005) *Wherever You Go There You Are: Mindfulness Meditation in Everyday Life*. Hyperion.

Pearson, J. C. (1992). *Lasting Love: What Keeps Couples Together*. William C. Brown.

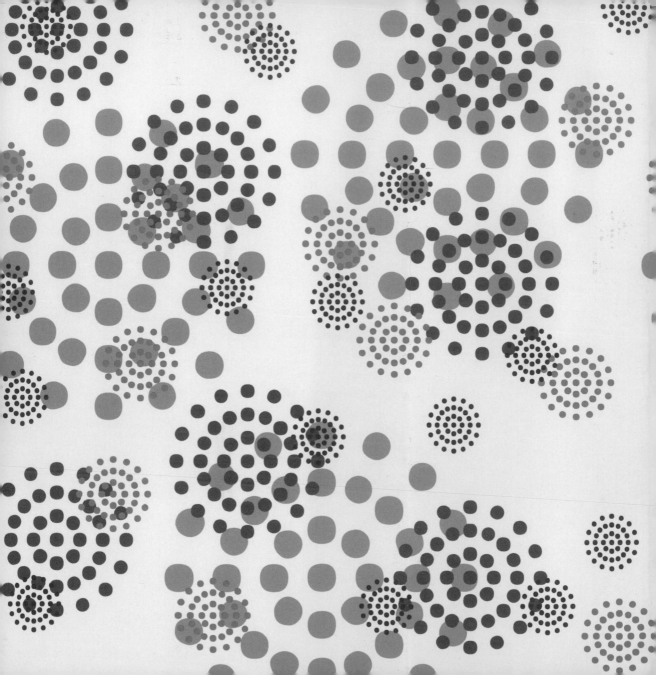